She Wears Lipstick to the Mailbox

Stop Hiding Behind Perfection. Heal Your Anxiety. Embrace Your True Self.

For every woman who looks fine on the outside but is falling apart on the inside.

Jan Truszkowski, MSW, LICSW

Still Standing: Anxiety Solutions Press
Wake Forest, NC

Copyright © 2025 Jan Truszkowski
All rights reserved.

No part of this publication may be reproduced, stored in a retrieval system, or transmitted in any form or by any means—electronic, mechanical, photocopying, recording, or otherwise—without the prior written permission of the author, except for brief quotations used in reviews or scholarly works.

This book is for educational and informational purposes only and is not intended as a substitute for individual mental health treatment. The author makes no guarantees regarding outcomes based on the use of this material.

Some names and identifying details have been changed to protect the privacy of individuals. Any resemblance to actual persons, living or dead, is purely coincidental.

Dedication

This book is dedicated to my husband, whom I love dearly—he supports me through all my craziness and never stops believing in me.

To my daughter, whom I love unconditionally and forever, and who loves me back—warts and all.

To my stepson and his wife, who are out in the world living and loving their big, beautiful lives.

To my two sisters and their husbands—my best friends—who have walked with me through so many chapters of life.

To my Greek sister-in-law, who will forever be family.

And to my creatively brilliant niece and her husband.

Finally, to all my clients, who inspired this book with their raw honesty and deep yearning to change their stories—to become more of who they were meant to be and to live happier, more fulfilling lives.

Preface

This book was born from a thousand therapy sessions and one beating heart—mine.

Over the years, I've worked with countless women who seemed to have it all together. They were smart, responsible, and endlessly giving. But beneath the surface, they were hurting. Not from anything obvious, but from a quiet kind of pain: emotional wounds left unhealed, needs left unmet, and lives spent performing instead of living.

Maybe that's you.

If you're tired of feeling anxious, burned out, invisible, or like no matter what you do, it's never enough—you're in the right place.

This isn't just a book to read. It's a companion for your healing.

Inside, you'll find:

- Therapist-guided reflections
- Real-life stories of transformation
- Journal prompts to help you uncover what's been buried
- Tools to shift the patterns that keep you stuck

I've woven in my own story, too—not because it's more important, but because healing is always easier when we don't feel alone.

This book won't tell you to work harder or think more positively. It will gently help you understand the emotional root of your suffering—and give you the tools to reclaim your sense of self, one page at a time.

The stories in this book are inspired by the real struggles and breakthroughs I've witnessed with my therapy clients. To honor their privacy, I've changed names, shifted details and combined experiences while illustrating their commonly shared issues. The case studies presented are camouflaged in such a way that no one individual's confidentiality would ever be revealed nor compromised.

So if you're ready to stop hiding behind perfection and start living with purpose, let's begin.

—Jan Truszkowski, MSW, LICSW

Table of Contents

Chapter 1: When Looking OK Matters More Than Being OK 1

Chapter 2: Where It All Began 7

Chapter 3: The Wounds of the Capable One 27

Chapter 4: Why You Can't Turn Off Your Mind 45

Chapter 5: Perfectionism and Control 67

Chapter 6: When Anxiety Becomes Identity 85

Chapter 7: The Inner Critic Isn't You 101

Chapter 8: Letting Go Without Falling Apart 121

Chapter 9: Self-Compassion, Rest, and Setting Boundaries 137

Chapter 10: You Were Never Broken 155

Afterword — What Happened To… 159

Acknowledgments 165

About the Author 167

Chapter 1:
When Looking OK Matters More Than Being OK

Are you a woman who's experienced chronic emotional pain?

You know the kind—that dull ache that never fully goes away. It might lift for a while, only to return like a heavy fog.

On the outside, you appear polished and put together.

On the inside, you're hurting. You're yearning. And you're constantly searching for relief.

Some women turn to alcohol or food. Some withdraw from the world. Some self-sabotage and take on a "bad" identity.

But this book is for the woman who copes by **doing**—the overfunctioner.

The one who stays busy to stay numb.

The one who is everything to everyone, but nothing to herself.

She puts her own needs last.

She blames herself when things go wrong—even when they aren't her fault.

She gives and gives, but never asks for help.

Do you know this woman?

Are you this woman?

Would you believe me if I told you that many of the struggles you're facing—anxiety, burnout, people-pleasing, perfectionism, self-doubt, even relationship difficulties—can often be traced back to a single source?

I know. It sounds too simple.

You're probably thinking:

"You're telling me all of my exhaustion and emotional pain come down to one thing?"

Yes. That's exactly what I'm saying.

And I'll show you how—and what you can do to finally feel better.

But first, let me tell you why I wrote this book.

As a therapist, I've sat across from hundreds of women who seemed to have it all together—smart, successful, capable. But underneath that polished exterior?

Exhaustion.

Anxiety.

Numbness.

Shame.

No matter what brought them into therapy—panic attacks, parenting struggles, career stress, or a vague sense of emptiness—our work often led to the same surprising truth:

There was a single emotional wound quietly shaping everything underneath.

Not the same wound for every woman—but always one core injury that had gone unacknowledged.

Sometimes it was rejection.

Sometimes abandonment.

Sometimes it was being silenced, unseen, unprotected, or made to believe that love had to be earned.

It would take weeks, sometimes months, to reach it. But when they did—often with tears—that's when the healing began.

I know this isn't just theory.

I lived it, too.

When I was four years old, my father died in a racing accident. His sudden death left a crater in my young world. I didn't understand grief, but I felt the absence of his love like a hole in my soul.

That was my wound: the loss of warmth, safety, and connection at the age I needed it most.

But my young brain couldn't process what had happened.

So I blamed myself.

I decided I must be bad. That's why Daddy left.

That belief burrowed deep.

Like many women, I grew up anxious, withdrawn, and unsure of myself—constantly trying to fill the invisible void inside. I had to be aloof to hide my flaws.

It wasn't until I stopped running from the pain—and turned to face it, name it, and grieve it—that I began to heal.

That's why I wrote this book.

To help women like you understand why you feel the way you do—and guide you gently toward healing what's been hurting for far too long.

My clients often say:

"This has been life-changing. I feel lighter now that I've stopped avoiding the truth."

That's what I want for you:

- Relief
- Healing
- Hope
- Joy
- Confidence
- Self-love

The heaviness you carry?

You weren't born with it.

You picked it up in a world that didn't always meet your needs.

But you don't have to carry it forever.
You weren't born to just function.

You were born to feel deeply, love fully, and live freely.

Let's begin your journey back to you.

This book will help you understand the link between your early emotional wounds and your adult anxiety. It offers therapy-informed tools, stories, and strategies to support your healing—and help you treat yourself with the compassion you've long given to others.

If you're the woman who's polished externally but crumbling internally, this book's for you. If you're the woman who wears lipstick, even to the mailbox, because appearing OK is more important than being OK, this book's for you.

So buckle up. I've got stories to tell—and healing to offer.

And maybe (just maybe), I'll make a few dollars to leave to my daughter, whom I love so dearly. ☺

Chapter 2:
Where It All Began

> "A mental wound is an unhealed injury
> and pain tied to the absence or loss of love."
> — Jan Truszkowski, MSW, LCSW, LICSW.

Would you believe me if I told you the pain running your life today likely started decades ago—not with the adult problems you can see, but with an injury you can't?

An invisible injury.

One that quietly altered the trajectory of your life.

You didn't choose it.

You didn't deserve it.

But it's there. And unless you recognize it, it will keep showing up—sabotaging your relationships, your peace, your decisions, even your sense of self.

We instinctively understand physical wounds:

You break a bone—you cast it.

You cut your skin—you clean and bandage it.

You sprain an ankle—you rest and protect it until it's strong again.

But what happens when the wound is invisible?

When it's emotional?

When no one even acknowledges it happened?

That's how an invisible injury begins.

And without attention, it doesn't heal. It festers. It grows.

It rewires the way you experience life—and not in your favor.

A Story About My Neighbor's Toe

When I was a kid, my neighbor—barefoot and carefree—sliced her big toe open on a jagged rock while playing in our yard. The cut was deep. Blood poured out. I knew if she walked home like that, the dirt and gravel would only make things worse. So I carried her.

Her mother, a nurse, took one look and sprang into action. She poured alcohol over the wound and scrubbed it clean. My friend screamed. Cried. Begged her to stop. But her mother didn't flinch—she disinfected it, bandaged it, and checked it daily.

Each time, my friend wailed in pain.

But because of that painful care, the wound healed—fully, cleanly, without lasting damage.

You might be thinking:

"Okay, but what does your friend's bloody toe have to do with my life being a mess?"

Well—imagine what would've happened if no one had cleaned the cut.

If she'd walked through dirt. Ignored the pain. Left it exposed.

Infection would have set in.

The pain would've gotten worse.

She wouldn't have been able to walk—missing out on her summer.

She would've been miserable, angry, hard to be around.

Eventually, she might have needed surgery—or worse.

"So... are you saying all my problems come from a cut toe?"

Not exactly.

But here's the truth:

An untreated wound—whether physical or emotional—doesn't just go away. It spreads.

It infects everything it touches. It alters how you live, how you move, how you see yourself and the world.

Why We Don't Heal

Most people never properly treat their deepest emotional wounds.

- They bandage them temporarily.
- They tell themselves to "move on."
- They power through.
- They stuff them down with food, alcohol, or drugs.

But the wound stays open—festering under the surface.

And over time, it quietly sabotages your happiness, your relationships, and your choices.

You can't build a thriving life on a festering wound.

You have to clean it.

You have to face the pain.

You have to heal.

And that's exactly what we're going to do together.

What Is a Mental Wound?

A mental wound is a deep emotional or psychological injury caused by experiences such as:

- Neglect
- Rejection
- Abuse

- Abandonment
- Betrayal
- Being chronically dismissed or invalidated

These wounds often form in childhood—sometimes through a single traumatic event, other times through repeated micro-injuries that build over time.

They may be invisible, but they're powerful.

They shape how you think, feel, behave, and relate to others.

Signs of an Untreated Mental Wound

- Chronic self-doubt
- Anxiety
- People-pleasing
- Emotional numbness
- Fear of intimacy
- Substance abuse
- Job instability
- A life that looks "fine" on the outside but feels empty inside

You might be suffering quietly—presenting a version of yourself to the world that's functional, but disconnected.

That mask protects you, but it also keeps you from being truly known.

The Essence of a Core Wound

At its root, a mental wound is unhealed injury and pain tied to the **absence or loss of love**.

- Sometimes that absence is active—like physical or emotional abuse.
- Sometimes it's passive—like neglect or emotional unavailability.
- And sometimes, it's loss—like the death of a parent or caregiver.

These experiences disrupt your sense of safety, belonging, and worth.

Left unhealed, they quietly dictate the direction of your life.

Heather's Story

Heather came into therapy after an emotional meltdown triggered by her sister canceling a visit. She cried uncontrollably, screamed, and felt emotionally unmoored for days. Her reaction was clearly disproportionate to the situation—her sister had simply felt overwhelmed and wasn't up to traveling.

Heather was both surprised and frightened by her own response. She feared she was "losing it."

As therapy progressed, the roots of her pain began to surface.

Heather's childhood had been chaotic—marked by abandonment and emotional neglect. Her mother, a nurse, worked long hours. Her father, a commercial fisherman, was often away for months at a time. As the youngest of three, Heather was mostly left to herself.

At age four, she broke her arm while unsupervised. Her siblings had left her alone, and her mother was at work. It was the third injury reported in three months, prompting a Child Protective Services investigation.

What was intended as a temporary placement became permanent when Heather and her siblings were placed in foster care. She remained there until she was emancipated at eighteen.

Heather's father showed little concern. He had another family and was emotionally checked out. Her mother, though she loved her children, was never able to pull her life together enough to care for them. Her own unhealed childhood trauma left her incapable of meeting even her own needs—let alone the needs of three children.

Heather's foster parents were emotionally distant and unkind. She never felt safe or loved in their care and often believed they were only in it for the money.

As an adult, Heather became emotionally shut down. She isolated herself, had no close friendships, no community, and no meaningful connections. She lived alone, emotionally flat, numb to joy or purpose. Her only contact was with others at her job, which she performed to perfection. She was fearful of making a mistake and being rejected. She agonized and ruminated if she made even the slightest, most non consequential mistake.

The canceled visit from her sister unearthed a deep emotional echo: the pain of being abandoned—again. Her reaction wasn't just about that day. It was about decades of unprocessed hurt that had never been acknowledged, named, or healed.

Heather's story is a powerful example of how unresolved emotional wounds can quietly shape the course of a life.

More on her story to follow…

Reflection Questions

You don't know what you don't know—which is kind of a problem when you're trying to live a healthy, balanced life. Most of us are so busy being productive, responsible, and emotionally available to *everyone* that we rarely stop to ask, "Wait... why am I doing this?" or "Do I even like this version of me?"

Therapists will tell you: change starts with awareness. And awareness starts with asking good questions—the kind that make you pause mid-scroll or mid-snack and go, "Oh wow... that hits."

All of the reflection questions in this book are here to help you hit that pause button. They're not tests. There are no wrong answers. Just small, meaningful prompts to help you get reacquainted with yourself—beneath the to-do lists, the lipstick, and the "I'm fine" face.

(Pro tip: Ask these to a close friend or partner over wine or coffee. Vulnerability and bonding almost guaranteed.)

WHERE IT ALL BEGAN

When you think back over your life, can you recall a painful memory that changed the trajectory of your life? Describe that memory in as much detail as possible including: what happened, your age, where you were and any details about your environment, who was present, how did others respond and behave, what were your thoughts about the incident, and what were the feelings you were experiencing. (Take your time and complete this question with as much detail as possible).

Perhaps you don't have just one memory but rather a series of memories with a common theme-such as being neglected or silenced or abused. Identify as many of those memories as you can including: what happened, your age, where you were and any details about your environment, who was present, how did others respond and behave, what were your thoughts about the incident, and what were the feelings you were experiencing. (Take your time and complete this question with as much detail as possible).

_____
_____
_____
_____
_____
_____
_____
_____
_____
_____
_____
_____
_____
_____
_____
_____
_____

Do you have a painful childhood memory that causes a lump in your throat or tears when you try to tell it? What is that memory and have you ever fully shared it with anyone? Why or why not? (Again, the more detail you can share the better).

If you've shared your painful childhood memories, what did it feel like to reveal your hurts? Did you feel exposed, raw, shame, guilt, sad, angry, relief, etc.? Describe your feelings in as much detail as possible. Bear in mind, you can experience more than one feeling at a time and your feelings can change.

_____
_____
_____
_____
_____
_____
_____
_____
_____
_____
_____
_____
_____
_____
_____
_____
_____
_____
_____

If you shared your painful memories, how did others respond to you? Did you get the reaction you'd hope for or were you disappointed in the response?

If you've never shared your painful childhood memories, why haven't you revealed the hurt you live with? What are you afraid of? What do think will happen if you share your pain?

Has your core wound affected you and your life in the following areas? If so, how?

Self-esteem
_____
_____
_____

Relationships
_____
_____
_____

Career
_____
_____
_____

Social Life
_____
_____
_____

Motivation
_____
_____
_____

In what ways have you tried to extinguish the constant pain you feel? Have your efforts worked or caused you more pain? If so, how?

What would it mean to you to no longer feel the constant invisible ache you've carried for so long? How would your life change?

Do you believe it's possible to cauterize your wound and contain the damage of your mental injury? If so, why? If not, why not?

If so, "Let's Do It".

If not, allow me to prove to you what's possible in the chapters ahead from my own experience and that of my clients.

Chapter 3:
The Wounds of the Capable One

"Sometimes the woman who seems to carry it all is the one most afraid to fall apart."

On the outside, Samantha's life looked successful. Inside, she was carrying the quiet cost of always being the "capable one."

Samantha's Story

Samantha was 37 years old, married, and the mother of three young children—ages 12, 8, and 7. She had worked hard to earn her law degree and held a demanding position at a criminal defense firm. Her long hours often meant missing family dinners. Her husband, a high school athletic director and football coach, was also frequently away from home.

Fortunately, they could afford help. They hired a loving, loyal, and energetic caretaker. The kids adored her. She cooked their favorite meals and filled their days with laughter and fun.

But despite the financial stability and professional success, Samantha was consumed by guilt and shame. She worried constantly about what her absence was doing to her children.

She came to therapy seeking relief from the crushing anxiety and guilt that followed her everywhere. She said she felt like she was "coming undone."

At night, after the house was quiet and everyone was asleep—including her husband—Samantha would binge on cookies, candy, ice cream, and chips.

She felt out of control. She hated the weight she had gained and carried deep shame about her eating habits.

She didn't understand why the urge to binge was so powerful. She just knew something wasn't right—and she needed help.

As she began to trust the therapy process, Samantha eventually shared a secret she had never told anyone. That secret—and how it shaped her sense of self—will be revealed later.

As you can see from Samantha's story, she was caught in an exhausting cycle. She felt enslaved to her work and her drive to achieve. In our sessions, she admitted she felt a compulsion to be the best attorney in her firm. She believed she had to bill the most hours, win the most cases, and never make a mistake.

At the same time, she deeply desired to give her children the best life she could. She provided them with every material advantage and had the support of a devoted nanny. Still, she was overwhelmed by guilt and shame.

She was always available at work. Always performing. But she was silently suffering.

There was an invisible pressure to "do it all"—and do it perfectly. That pressure was suffocating. It was snuffing out her light. She was robotically going through the motions of someone who *has it all*—but inside, she was slowly dying. And no one knew.

You'll learn what happened to Samantha later.

Maybe your life doesn't look exactly like Samantha's.

Maybe you don't have a high-powered career or a nanny to help with the kids.

Maybe you're a stay-at-home mom juggling volunteer work, school drop-offs, athletic practices, and countless to-do lists.

Maybe you're the one who remembers every birthday, plans every celebration, schedules every appointment, and keeps everything running smoothly.

Maybe you're caring for a child with special needs, or an aging parent who depends on you.

Regardless of the specifics, you may know exactly what Samantha feels:

That invisible pressure to be everything to everyone.

That guilt that whispers you're still not doing enough.

That inner voice that tells you—*no matter how much you do, it's not good enough.*

Tip Box

Signs You Might Be "The Capable One"

- You're the one people come to when they need help, advice, or a favor
- You rarely ask for help—even when you're struggling
- You often feel like you don't have the "luxury" of falling apart
- You feel guilty when you rest or say no
- You're praised for being strong, organized, reliable, or selfless

- You put others' needs ahead of your own—almost automatically
- You silently manage the details no one else sees (schedules, emotions, crises)
- You minimize your pain because "other people have it worse"
- You keep your feelings to yourself so you won't be a burden
- You push through exhaustion, overwhelm, or illness because you "have to"
- You feel like everything would fall apart if you stopped holding it all together

Exercise: How to Begin Letting Go of Over-Functioning

1. Start Noticing, Without Judgment
Awareness is the first step. Begin to observe the moments when you jump in to solve, fix, soothe, or manage. Ask yourself, *"Is this truly mine to carry?"*

2. Practice the Pause
Before saying yes, rescuing, or volunteering, take a breath. Try responding with, "Let me get back to you," to give yourself space to consider *your* needs.

3. Build Tolerance for Discomfort
Over-functioning often masks a fear of being seen as lazy, selfish, or "not enough." Remind yourself that rest is not weakness—and discomfort doesn't mean danger.

4. Delegate Without Apology
Start small. Ask for help with something you'd normally take on alone. Resist the urge to micromanage the outcome. Let it be "good enough."

5. Redefine What It Means to Be Strong

True strength isn't doing it all—it's knowing your limits, honoring your needs, and allowing others to rise to the occasion.

6. Make Space for Receiving

Let someone care for *you*. Whether it's accepting a compliment, a helping hand, or emotional support—practice softening into the unfamiliar act of receiving.

7. Rewrite the Old Story

Journal a new narrative: *"I am not responsible for holding everything together. I can rest. I can trust others. I can still be loved when I'm not performing."*

Reflection Questions: Recognizing Over-Functioning and Self-Neglect

When something goes wrong in your family, workplace, or relationships, do you immediately feel it's your job to fix it? Why do you think that is?

_____
_____
_____
_____
_____
_____
_____
_____
_____
_____
_____
_____
_____
_____
_____
_____
_____
_____
_____
_____
_____
_____
_____
_____

Do you ever feel resentful or exhausted but keep pushing through because "there's no one else to do it"? What would happen if you stopped?

How comfortable are you letting others take the lead or handle something without your involvement? What thoughts or emotions come up when you try?

_____
_____
_____
_____
_____
_____
_____
_____
_____
_____
_____
_____
_____
_____
_____
_____
_____
_____
_____
_____
_____

Have you been praised or valued more for what you *do* than for who you *are*? How might that affect how you see your worth today?

Do you find it difficult to ask for help—even when you truly need it? What beliefs hold you back from reaching out?

When was the last time you made a decision based purely on *your own* needs or desires, without factoring in everyone else's? How did it feel?

In your close relationships, do you often carry the emotional load—keeping the peace, checking in, remembering birthdays, solving conflicts? How does that impact your energy?

If you stopped being the reliable one, the helper, or the strong one, who might you fear disappointing—or who might you fear becoming?

Do you equate rest or relaxation with laziness or guilt? What internal messages drive that belief?

What would change in your life if you believed it was safe to need, safe to receive, and safe to let go?

Digging Deeper Exercise: Releasing the Weight You Carry
"What I Hold vs. What I Can Let Go"

Step 1: List the Weight You Carry
Take a quiet moment and complete the following sentence starters in your journal:

- I feel responsible for...
- People count on me to...
- If I don't do it, then...
- I worry that if I stop helping, then...

Let yourself write freely. Don't censor or edit—just notice what comes up.

Step 2: Identify the Hidden Belief
Now look at your list. Underneath each responsibility or fear, ask yourself:

- What belief might be driving this?

(e.g., "If I'm not needed, I'm not valuable," or "If I don't do it perfectly, I'll be rejected.")

Write those beliefs down next to each item.

Step 3: Challenge the Old Narrative
Choose one or two of those beliefs and journal your response to this question:

- Where did I learn this belief? Is it still serving me today?

Then write a **new belief** to replace it.

Examples:

- "I am worthy of rest."
- "Being loved does not require overextending myself."

Step 4: Practice Letting Go
Create two columns titled:

"What I Choose to Keep" | "What I Can Begin to Let Go"

Fill in each side with intention. For example:

Keep: Being emotionally available to my children

Let Go: Fixing every problem before they even ask for help

Step 5: Affirmation for Healing
Close your entry by writing this (or your own version) in bold:

"I no longer have to prove my worth through exhaustion. I am allowed to rest, receive, and just be me."

Chapter 4:
Why You Can't Turn Off Your Mind

"My mind's like a browser with 50 tabs open, and none of them are loading."

You lie in bed exhausted, but your mind is still wide awake—running through worst-case scenarios, replaying a conversation from three days ago, or mentally rewriting your to-do list for the hundredth time.

You tell yourself to relax. You try breathing exercises. You even count sheep. But still, the thoughts won't stop.

Why does your mind keep doing this?

You're not broken.

You're not failing.

Your mind is trying to *protect* you.

Let's look at how—and why—this relentless mental noise develops, starting with Angela's story.

Angela's Story: On the Surface

Angela was a married, accomplished dentist in her thirties, expecting her first child. Her life looked picture-perfect—financially stable, married to a man she loved, and eagerly preparing for motherhood.

Yet beneath the surface, Angela was plagued by relentless anxiety.

She worried about everything—whether she was gaining too much weight during pregnancy, whether the baby would be healthy, whether the nursery furniture had been properly assembled. Her mind was like a hamster wheel—constantly turning, never resting.

Overthinking as a Form of Protection

Overthinking often feels like problem-solving—but it's actually your brain's attempt to **control uncertainty** and **prevent emotional pain**.

Angela's mind was constantly scanning for danger. Why? Because danger had been real for her.

As a child, the consequences of not anticipating her mother's moods could result in violence.

So her brain learned: *If I worry about every possible outcome, maybe I can prevent something bad from happening.*

This is called **anticipatory anxiety**—a type of anxiety that arises not from current danger, but from imagined future threats.

The overthinking isn't random. It's your brain trying to predict and prevent harm. But instead of bringing peace, it creates more suffering.

Angela's Story: The Impostor Within

Angela's anxiety wasn't limited to her personal life. At work, it was just as intense.

Despite her advanced degree and years of positive feedback, she was haunted by a fear of being exposed as a fraud.

This is **Impostor Syndrome**—the persistent belief that you're not as competent as others think you are, and that eventually, you'll be "found out."

To cope, Angela worked late hours, checking and rechecking her dental work. This soothed her anxiety temporarily, but it created tension with her staff and reinforced the belief that her work needed to be *perfect* in order to be acceptable.

Angela's inner critic was brutal. It whispered:

- "You're going to mess up."
- "They're going to see you don't belong."
- "You're a disappointment."

Even though there was no evidence for these beliefs, Angela clung to them—because they *felt* true.

Cognitive Distortions: The Lies Your Mind Tells

Cognitive distortions are distorted patterns of thinking that make us feel anxious, unworthy, or stuck.

They're not based on fact—but on fear, learned beliefs, and emotional memory.

Some common distortions Angela struggled with:

- **Catastrophizing:** Expecting the worst-case scenario ("What if the baby dies?")
- **All-or-nothing thinking:** "If I don't do this perfectly, I'm a failure."
- **Mind reading:** "My staff thinks I'm incompetent."
- **Personalization:** "If something goes wrong, it must be my fault."

These distortions formed not because Angela was irrational—but because they once served a purpose: they helped her make sense of a chaotic world. They were her brain's way of creating order in the emotional chaos of childhood.

Tip Box: 5 Common Cognitive Distortions That Keep You Stuck

When your mind won't turn off, chances are you're caught in one or more of these distorted thinking patterns. These are *automatic* and *learned*—you didn't choose them, but you can learn to recognize and challenge them.

1. Catastrophizing

Jumping to the worst-case scenario—even when there's little or no evidence it will happen.

"If I make a mistake at work, I'll lose my job. Then we'll lose the house. Then..."

* This distortion keeps your nervous system in a state of constant emergency.

2. All-or-Nothing Thinking

Seeing things in black-and-white terms, with no room for nuance.

"If I don't do this perfectly, I'm a complete failure."

* This mindset leads to chronic self-judgment and perfectionism.

3. Mind Reading

Assuming you know what others are thinking—usually something negative about you.

"They think I'm incompetent."

* It creates unnecessary anxiety and undermines your self-confidence.

4. Personalization

Blaming yourself for things outside your control—or assuming everything is your fault.

"She's upset. It must be something I did."

* This distortion can stem from early caregiving environments where you felt responsible for other people's emotions.

5. Should Statements

Rigid rules you place on yourself or others, often leading to guilt or frustration.

"I should be able to handle this better."

* These "shoulds" are often internalized from caregivers, culture, or past expectations—and rarely allow room for grace.

✓ What to Do:

- Start *noticing* when these distortions show up in your thoughts.
- Ask: "Is this thought absolutely true? Or could there be another explanation?"
- Talk to yourself the way you'd talk to a beloved friend—not a harsh critic.

Angela's Story: A Glimpse Into Childhood

To understand why Angela's mind couldn't stop scanning for danger, we had to look backward.

Angela was the oldest of four children. Her father was kind, but often absent. Her mother was physically and emotionally abusive—especially to Angela, who tried to protect her younger siblings and became the main target of her mother's rage.

Her mother's anger was terrifying and calculated. It only happened when her father was away. Angela quickly learned: *You are never safe. You have to be on guard. Always.*

Angela didn't just develop anxiety—she developed **hypervigilance**. Her nervous system became conditioned to stay in a **constant state of readiness**. Her body was living in the past, expecting the next emotional ambush—even in her adult life.

The Fight, Flight, or Freeze Trap

When you live in chronic fear or uncertainty, your nervous system gets stuck in a survival loop: **fight, flight, or freeze**.

- **Fight** might look like perfectionism or controlling behavior.
- **Flight** might look like avoiding confrontation or being constantly busy.
- **Freeze** might look like emotional shutdown, indecision, or numbing.

Angela's fight mode showed up as over-preparing, controlling her environment, and striving for flawless work.

Her flight response showed up as people-pleasing and conflict avoidance.

When overwhelmed, she froze—doubting herself, shutting down emotionally, and feeling stuck.

These were not conscious choices. They were adaptive responses—rooted in trauma and shaped by survival.

Angela's Story: The Breaking Point

One day, during her teenage years, Angela's mother struck her in the face, leaving a visible bruise.

Angela told her father she had fallen into the coffee table while dancing.

But her visiting aunt wasn't convinced.

While shopping later that day, her aunt gently asked, "Did your mother hit you?"

For the first time, Angela broke. Overwhelmed with emotion, she told the truth.

That moment marked the beginning of a new chapter—one where Angela no longer had to carry the secret alone.

The Takeaway: You Are Not Broken—You Are Wired for Survival

If your mind is always racing…

If you struggle to sleep, to slow down, or to feel safe in stillness…

It's not because something is wrong with you.

It's because something *happened* to you.

Your brain and body adapted to survive what you lived through.

Your overthinking isn't just noise—it's a shield.

Your anxiety isn't weakness—it's a warning system that was programmed by pain.

Your inner critic isn't cruelty—it's a misguided protector trying to keep you from harm.

It's because your nervous system—and your inner world—never had the chance to fully feel safe.

Overthinking, anxiety, impostor syndrome—they're all responses to pain.

They're not who you are. They're survival strategies.

But survival is only the beginning.

You're not a little girl hiding in fear anymore.

You're an adult with access to compassion, truth, and healing.

This chapter wasn't about diagnosing you—it was about helping you *understand* you.

When we understand our symptoms, we begin to loosen their grip.

We begin to see our thoughts not as enemies, but as echoes—calling for attention, care, and restoration.

You don't have to keep living in mental overdrive.

You can learn to feel safe again—not just in your environment, but in your own mind.
And that, dear reader, is what healing begins to look like.

Reflection Questions: Why You Can't Turn Off Your Mind

What parts of Angela's life seem most stable or secure on the outside?

What parts of your own life might look "fine" to others, even if they don't feel that way inside?

Have you ever felt anxious even when everything "looked good" in your life?

What did that experience reveal about your inner world?

What does it feel like to be stuck in a loop of "what if" thinking?
How does your body respond in those moments? How do you usually cope?

When you feel like an impostor, what specific fears come up for you?
Are they rooted in fact, or in old emotional patterns?

How does your "inner critic" keep you stuck in doubt—even when there's no real evidence?
What is that critical voice trying to protect you from?

What is one way you might begin to challenge that impostor voice?

What would a more truthful and compassionate voice sound like?

How does Angela's childhood experience help explain her anxiety in adulthood?
What early life experiences may have shaped your own inner world?

In what ways did Angela learn to hide her pain and protect others?

Have you ever taken on a similar role? At what cost to yourself?

Have you ever felt the need to protect others at your own expense?
What did you gain or lose by doing so?

How did Angela's secret-keeping impact her adult life?
Are there any secrets or unspoken truths you still carry today?

When has it been difficult for you to speak your truth—even when someone asked directly?
What held you back? What did you fear?

What did it feel like (or what might it feel like) to finally admit the truth to someone safe?

How might your life change if you allowed yourself to be truly known?

Chapter 5:
Perfectionism and Control

"I don't have a problem with control—I just think everything would be better if I did it myself... exactly the right way."

You're constantly trying to get it right.

To say the right thing.

To look the right way.

To avoid mistakes, criticism, or failure—at all costs.

Maybe you overprepare, overthink, overwork.

Or maybe you shut down entirely, afraid that if you can't do it perfectly, it's better not to try.

Underneath perfectionism and the need for control is not pride—it's pain.

A fear of rejection.

A fear of shame.

A fear that if you let your guard down, you'll be exposed, hurt, or abandoned.

Perfectionism doesn't mean you think you're better than everyone else.

It often means you feel *not good enough* at your core—and you're trying to earn your right to exist without being hurt again.

Control as a Trauma Response

Children don't get to control their environment. But when things are painful, unpredictable, or chaotic, many learn to control themselves instead.

They become hypervigilant—scanning for signs of danger.

They become responsible—always doing the "right" thing.

They try to be invisible—or perfect—to avoid punishment or disapproval.

Control becomes a way to survive.

It gives the illusion of safety:

- *"If I don't make a mistake, I won't be shamed."*
- *"If I take care of everything, no one can be mad at me."*
- *"If I do it all right, maybe I'll finally feel enough."*

But control is exhausting. And perfection is a moving target.

No matter how much you do, the fear remains.

Because what you're really trying to control is not just your outer world—but the inner fear that you're not enough.

Lea's Story

Lea came to therapy after she began having panic attacks. They would strike without warning—one moment she was fine, and the next she was consumed by a terrifying sense of dread. At first, she thought she was dying. Then came the fear of the fear itself. The panic began to control her.

Her world shrank quickly. She stopped going out with friends. Stopped going to the gym. Stopped driving beyond familiar roads. Her once-full life became small and tightly contained.

On the surface, Lea had always been a high achiever. In childhood, while other kids played after school, Lea studied. She earned straight A's and soaked up the praise that followed. As an adult, she became the Marketing Director at a successful tech startup. Her campaigns won awards. She regularly received bonuses. People admired her dedication.

But inside, she was unraveling.

As trust deepened in therapy, Lea shared a pivotal memory. When she was seven, her mother left the family—just one day after Lea's birthday party. Her parents had argued the night before, and though she couldn't understand what was said, she remembered hearing her mother say her name. And then she was gone.

Lea's young mind drew one conclusion: *It was my fault.*

That single belief took root and shaped everything that followed. If she could just be perfect—good enough, successful enough, composed enough—maybe no one would ever leave her again.

Her perfectionism wasn't arrogance. It was armor.

A strategy to survive heartbreak she never should have had to carry.

But eventually, the cost became too high: chronic stomach issues, sleepless nights, a racing mind that never rested, and finally, panic attacks that forced her to confront the truth—

She didn't feel safe unless she was performing.

Doing It Right to Stay Safe

Perfectionism isn't always about neatness or achievement. Sometimes it shows up as:

- Being the fixer in your relationships
- Avoiding vulnerability
- Silencing your real feelings
- Believing love has to be earned

If you were taught that mistakes made you bad or unlovable, then being "good" becomes your shield.

But the problem with using perfectionism as protection is that it also cuts you off from real connection.

Because when you're performing, you're not being seen.

You're managing perception—not living freely.

Lea tried to manage how others saw her—driven, competent, unshakable.

But underneath, she was still the little girl who believed she had to be perfect to be loved.

The Cost of Control

Control often starts as protection—but it eventually becomes a prison.

It keeps you from taking risks or being creative.

It robs you of spontaneity and joy.

It keeps you in a constant state of self-monitoring and shame.

Worst of all, it reinforces the belief that you are only safe when you are perfect.

Lea's healing began when she started telling the truth—not just about what happened to her, but about the painful beliefs she carried into adulthood.

She came to understand:

Her behaviors weren't flaws. They were coping mechanisms.

And while control once kept her safe, it was now keeping her stuck.

You may have learned that being in control protected you.

But healing begins when you realize: you don't have to earn your worth anymore.

Tip Box: How to Spot When Control Is Running the Show

Control isn't always obvious. It doesn't always look like being bossy or rigid.

Sometimes it's quiet, disguised as responsibility, planning, or even being "the strong one."

Here are subtle signs that control may be leading your life—not love, not trust, not peace:

1. You struggle to delegate.
You tell yourself, "It's just easier if I do it myself," but underneath that is a fear that things will fall apart—or reflect badly on you—if you let go.

2. You over-prepare for everything.
You spend excessive time anticipating every possible outcome, conversation, or scenario so nothing catches you off guard.

3. You feel anxious when things are unplanned or uncertain.
Spontaneity feels unsafe, not exciting. You feel panicked when things don't go "just right."

4. You keep emotions tightly locked away.
You don't want to burden others. Vulnerability feels like losing control, so you keep it together—even when you're breaking inside.

5. You tie your worth to performance.
You only feel good about yourself when you're achieving, succeeding, helping, or fixing. If you're not doing something productive, you feel unworthy.

6. You avoid asking for help.
Letting others show up for you feels uncomfortable—or even shameful. You equate independence with safety.

7. You micromanage people, conversations, or emotions.

Even in relationships, you try to manage how others feel, respond, or behave—because it helps you feel secure.

A Gentle Reminder:

Control is not who you are—it's how you learned to feel safe.

You don't have to earn rest. You don't have to prove your worth.

You are allowed to exhale, even when life is still uncertain.

Reflection Questions: Perfectionism and Control

What situations make you feel the need to have everything "just right" before moving forward, and what fears (e.g., failure, criticism, or rejection) might be driving this need?

How often do you find yourself over-preparing or obsessing over details to ensure others approve of your work or actions? What happens when things don't go as planned?

When faced with uncertainty or ambiguity, do you notice yourself trying to control outcomes (e.g., planning excessively, —seeking reassurance)? What emotions come up when you can't control the situation?

How do you react when someone points out a mistake or flaw in your work? Does the fear of being judged or rejected influence your response?

Are there times when you avoid starting or completing tasks because you're worried they won't meet your own high standards? What thoughts or feelings arise in those moments?

Do you often feel responsible for how others perceive you or for their emotional reactions? How does this lead to controlling behaviors or perfectionist tendencies?

How do you handle situations where you might not be in full control (e.g., group projects, unpredictable events)? Does anxiety or fear of rejection surface, and how do you cope?

Reflect on a recent time you felt anxious or rejected. Did you respond by trying to perfect something (e.g., your appearance, work, or behavior) or by trying to control the situation? Why?

Do you find yourself seeking constant validation or approval from others to feel secure? How does this connect to your efforts to avoid mistakes or imperfections?

What would it feel like to let go of the need to be perfect or in control in a specific situation? What fears or anxieties come up when you imagine this?

Chapter 6:
When Anxiety Becomes Identity

*"My anxiety is so attached to me,
it might as well get its own seat at the table."*

You weren't born anxious.

You became anxious in response to something.

Maybe it was chaos, criticism, emotional absence, or the unspoken expectation that your needs were too much.

Maybe it was subtle. Or maybe it was sharp and obvious.

Either way, anxiety often begins as a way to stay safe.

To scan for danger.

To prepare for disappointment.

To try and prevent pain.

But over time, anxiety stops being something you *experience*—and becomes someone you *believe you are*.

It becomes fused with your identity:

"I'm just an anxious person."

"I'm a mess."

"I'm always the one who worries."

"I'm the one who can't get it together."

But anxiety isn't who you are.

It's a response.

A protector.

A set of patterns that once kept you safe—and now keep you stuck.

The Roles We Inherit

When you grow up in a family system where emotional needs are unmet, unacknowledged, or punished, children adapt by taking on roles to survive:

- The Peacemaker
- The Overachiever
- The Black Sheep
- The Caretaker
- The Invisible One
- The Clown

These roles help make sense of the chaos. They offer identity, direction, and sometimes even attention or approval.

But these roles are not based on who you are at your core—they're based on what was needed to survive.

Blair's Story: Becoming the "Bad" One

Blair first entered therapy after being fired for stealing from her employer. She acted like it didn't matter much, brushing it off with sarcasm and defiance. She only agreed to therapy because her partner insisted.

But underneath her bravado was a deep well of shame.

Blair was the oldest of two daughters. Her younger sister was everything her mother wanted: compliant, soft-spoken, and easy to manage. Blair, on the other hand, was outspoken, bold, and unwilling to play small. She was told she was too much—too loud, too wild, too difficult to love.

When Blair tried to speak up about the obvious favoritism in the home, her mother dismissed her, turning the blame back on Blair: *"You're the one who causes problems."*

Her father, though he saw the dynamic, stayed silent.

Over time, Blair began to believe what was reflected back to her:

That she was bad.

That she was a disappointment.

That she didn't belong.

So she embraced the identity she was given.

If she was going to be the "bad one," she figured, she might as well *be* bad.

She rebelled.

She plagiarized.

She stole.

She self-sabotaged.

Her anxiety—though masked by anger and indifference—was constant. She lived in fight-or-flight, her nervous system stuck in survival mode. The only control she had was to act before others could hurt or reject her again.

The black sheep identity became a self-fulfilling prophecy.

A Return to Samantha's Story: The "Best" One

While Blair coped by being the rebel, *Samantha* coped by being perfect.

As you recall, she was the high-achieving criminal defense attorney and mother of three, Samantha spent her life trying to be everything to everyone. She stayed late at the office to make sure she was the "best" attorney in the firm. Although she had the help of a Nanny, she still felt responsibility for making sure all of her family's needs were met. She pushed herself beyond exhaustion, believing it was her responsibility to hold everything—and everyone—together.

Samantha's accomplishments became the way she received love and approval. Over time, her identity became fused with productivity and perfection.

"I'm the strong one."

"I can handle it."

"I don't have needs."

But underneath her success was crushing anxiety—guilt, overwhelm, and the constant fear of letting people down.

Samantha's identity was not rooted in who she truly was, but in the role she played for survival: *the responsible one.*

She didn't know who she was apart from what she could *do*.

When Roles Become Identity

Whether you became the "bad one" or the "best one," the pain is the same:

Your true self was buried beneath a performance—either for attention, protection, or survival.

You learned that who you were wasn't acceptable or safe. So you adapted.

But what helped you survive as a child may now be causing anxiety in adulthood:

- If you were the *fixer*, you may now feel panic if people are upset or unwell.
- If you were the *overachiever*, rest may feel like failure.
- If you were the *scapegoat*, self-sabotage might feel familiar and even strangely safe.

You may not even realize you're living from a role, because it feels so fused with your personality.

But here's the truth:

You are not your anxiety.

You are not your productivity.

You are not the problem.

You are not the performance.

You are someone who learned how to survive.

Now you get to learn how to be free.

Tip Box: Signs Your Anxiety Has Become Your Identity

- You say things like "I'm just a worrier" or "That's just who I am"
- You feel guilt or shame when you're not being productive
- You don't know who you are apart from your roles (mom, worker, helper, achiever)
- You define yourself by your mistakes or failures
- You feel unsafe resting, relaxing, or letting your guard down
- You sabotage things that go well because it feels unfamiliar
- You struggle to imagine a version of yourself that isn't anxious

A Gentle Reminder:

The roles you played were never a reflection of your worth.

They were coping strategies—nothing more.

You're allowed to grow beyond them.

You're allowed to heal.

You're allowed to become who you really are—without performance, without apology.

Reflection Questions: When Anxiety Becomes Identity

How do I describe myself when I think about my anxiety?

(For example: "I am always anxious," or "I can never relax.")

In what ways do I find myself using anxiety as a way to explain my actions or decisions?

(For example: "I can't do that because I'm too anxious," or "I always worry before doing something new.")

What thoughts or beliefs about myself seem to be rooted in anxiety?
(Consider: "I'm not good enough," or "I can't handle stress.")

How often do I identify myself with the feeling of anxiety, as opposed to recognizing it as something I experience but not who I am?

When was the last time I noticed anxiety dictating my choices or limiting my actions? What happened in that moment?

If I took anxiety out of my life for a moment, how would I describe myself differently? What would I be able to do that I feel is impossible now?

What labels or phrases do I use to define myself in relation to my anxiety (e.g., "I am a worrier," or "I am always on edge")?

How do I feel when I try to step outside my comfort zone and push past anxiety? Does it feel like I'm resisting a part of myself?

What would it look like for me to release my attachment to anxiety as part of my identity? How would I behave differently?

What are some moments in my life where I've been able to find peace or calm despite my anxiety? How can I remind myself that anxiety doesn't define me during those moments?

Chapter 7:
The Inner Critic Isn't You

"The inner critic is just a scared echo of your past—not the voice of your truth. You don't have to believe everything it says to you."

You hear it in your head.

That voice that whispers—or shouts—that you're not good enough.

That you'll mess it up. That you'll be rejected. That you'll never be loved the way you long to be.

It sounds like truth.

But it isn't.

The inner critic is not your true voice.

It's the echo of pain.

The internalized voice of people who didn't see you, love you, or protect you the way you deserved.

It's the distorted belief you absorbed as a child and never had the tools—or permission—to question.

You were not born thinking you were bad, broken, or unworthy.

You learned it.

And anything learned can be unlearned.

How the Brain Works When Perpetuating Lies About Yourself

Neuroscience helps explain why we hold onto painful beliefs long after they've outlived their usefulness. Our brains are wired for survival, not truth. Once we internalize a belief—especially in childhood—it becomes a sort of mental shortcut. The brain begins filtering all new experiences through that belief, looking for consistency.

And because the brain favors familiarity, it holds onto painful thoughts simply because they feel "known."

My Story: When the Inner Critic Was Born

I grew up in the beautiful foothills of North Carolina. My mother was a devoted homemaker who loved her family and enjoyed cooking, dancing, gardening, and all things sports. My father was one of the early pioneers of NASCAR—racing cars, hauling moonshine, and eventually co-owning the North Wilkesboro Speedway.

From the outside, it looked like an idyllic life. But in March of 1958, when I was just four years old, everything changed.

My father died in a racing accident.

My mother had given birth to my baby brother only eleven days earlier. My two older sisters were five and twelve years old. When my uncle showed up at our house before the race had even ended, my mother fainted on sight.

She knew instantly. My uncle was there to tell us that my father's car had flipped and pinned him beneath it. He didn't survive.

As a four-year-old, I couldn't grasp what had happened. I was lifted to peer over the edge of the "box" where my father lay at the funeral. He wasn't wearing his usual grease-covered overalls but a navy jacket and tie, resting on a silky white pillow. I thought he was just sleeping and might pop up like a jack-in-the-box.

But something inside me shifted.

I was too young to understand death—but old enough to form a thought: *He's gone. I must have done something bad.*

That thought fused with overwhelming emotion—grief, confusion, abandonment—and became a belief: *I am bad.*

That belief became my inner critic's voice.

And that voice shaped everything.

I began to build armor—not visible armor, but emotional protection.

I withdrew, acted out, pushed people away.

If someone liked me, I didn't trust it. That contradicted the story in my head. So I'd behave in ways that would confirm the "truth" I believed: that I wasn't lovable, that I was broken.

And when people pulled away, I used it as more proof.

I created the very rejection I feared.

Not because I wanted to—but because I was trying to survive with a belief that never should have been mine.

Why Facts Don't Always Change Feelings

Even when people praised me, it didn't register. Compliments felt suspicious.

If someone saw something good in me, my brain whispered: *They don't really know me.*

This is a common experience for those with early emotional wounds. When you've internalized shame or inadequacy, your brain is wired to reject anything that challenges that belief.

Reflection: Dismissing the Positive
- Have you ever dismissed a compliment or positive feedback? What did you think or feel?
- Have you experienced a conflict between how others see you and how you see yourself?
- What do you typically tell yourself when someone offers praise or kindness?

Confirmation Bias: Seeing What We Already Believe

The brain's confirmation bias ensures that once we believe something—especially about ourselves—we unconsciously seek out "proof" that it's true.

We magnify negative feedback and minimize the positive.

We remember the times we failed and forget the times we succeeded.

This kept me trapped in a loop. I looked for evidence I was "bad."

Every rejection, every misstep, every silence became proof.

Reflection: Searching for "Proof"
- What belief about yourself do you often seek to confirm, even unconsciously?
- How do you respond when something challenges that belief?
- Do you ever distort or dismiss positive experiences to fit your inner story?

When Behavior Reinforces the Lie

When you believe you're bad, broken, or unworthy, your actions often reflect that.

Not consciously—but subtly. Through self-sabotage, avoidance, isolation, or overcompensation-such as perfectionism.

I did things that pushed people away.

I retreated into silence or acted out.

It was all a way to regulate the unbearable tension between what others saw and what I believed about myself.

Reflection: Acting Out the Story
- Have you ever behaved in a way that confirmed a painful belief about yourself?

- What role has shame or self-judgment played in your decisions or relationships?
- What might be different if you no longer felt the need to "prove" your unworthiness?

The Armor You Built

Like me, you didn't set out to build armor—you just wanted to feel safe.

When love disappeared, when loss came too soon, when your feelings were ignored or punished, you adapted. You created strategies to survive:

- Perfectionism
- People-pleasing
- Numbing
- Control
- Overachievement
- Withdrawal
- Defiance
- Sarcasm
- Independence that kept everyone at arm's length

These weren't flaws. They were protective mechanisms.

And they worked—for a while.

When Protection Becomes a Prison

Eventually, that armor—meant to shield you—starts to trap you.

You're exhausted from over-functioning.

You can't rest without guilt.

You avoid intimacy because it feels too risky.

You stay quiet because speaking up feels dangerous.

You sabotage closeness because it challenges your story.

This is the cost of the inner critic's reign.

It keeps pain out, but it keeps love out, too.

It numbs your fear—but also your joy.

But here's the truth:

The inner critic is not you. It's the voice of a wound, not your wisdom.

Power Up Your Thoughts

The inner critic is not your true self.

It's the scared child who absorbed a false story and has been trying to make sense of pain ever since.

But you are no longer that child.

You have words now. Tools. Awareness. And a choice.

You can choose to listen to a kinder voice.

You can rewrite the narrative.

And you can lay down the armor.

Because you were never the problem.

You were always worthy—just waiting to believe it.

Exercise: Name Your Inner Critic
Naming your inner critic can be a powerful way to externalize the negative voice inside your head, making it feel less personal and easier to challenge. Here are some reasons why giving your inner critic a name might be beneficial:

Reasons to Name Your Inner Critic:

1. **Creates Distance**: Naming your inner critic helps you separate yourself from the negative voice. Instead of thinking "I am not good enough," you might think "Oh, that's just *Whiny Wendy* talking again."
2. **Reduces Its Power**: Giving the critic a funny or silly name can make it seem less intimidating. It's hard to take negative thoughts seriously when they're coming from *Tattle-Tale Tina*.
3. **Makes It Easier to Challenge**: When you give your inner critic a name, it becomes easier to talk back. Instead of just "shutting it down," you can imagine having a conversation with this character.
4. **Humor Helps**: Humor is a great tool for reducing anxiety and making difficult situations feel more manageable. Laughing at your inner critic can neutralize its sting.
5. **Helps With Emotional Detachment**: Naming your critic allows you to see it as something external rather than internal, reducing the emotional impact of its harsh words.
6. **Increases Awareness**: Naming your inner critic encourages you to become more aware of when it's speaking, helping you notice the patterns and trigger points more easily.

Funny Name Ideas for Your Inner Critic:

1. Negative Nancy
2. Debbie Downer
3. Whiny Wendy
4. Perfectionist Paula
5. Judgmental Jill
6. Fearful Fiona
7. Gloomy Gia
8. Critical Cruella

By giving your inner critic a playful or exaggerated name, you can soften its impact and reduce its ability to dominate your thoughts. You can also make the inner critic feel less powerful by imagining how you'd handle it if it were a real person – with humor, compassion, and confidence!

Reflection Questions: Rewriting the Inner Narrative

What are the most common things my inner critic tells me about myself?

(For example: "You're not good enough," "You'll never succeed.")

_____
_____
_____
_____
_____
_____
_____
_____
_____
_____
_____
_____
_____
_____
_____
_____
_____
_____
_____

When I make a mistake, what does my inner critic say?

(Consider: "You should've known better," or "You always mess up.")

How does my inner critic speak to me in times of stress or anxiety?
(For example: "You're failing," or "Everyone is judging you.")

What phrases or words does my inner critic use to make me feel small or unworthy?
(Look for recurring language like "never," "always," or "too much.")

In what areas of my life do I hear my inner critic the loudest?
(Is it work, relationships, body image, or other aspects of life?)

What would I say to a friend if they were talking to themselves the way my inner critic talks to me?

(Write a compassionate response to yourself as if you were comforting a friend.)

How does my inner critic affect my behavior?
(Does it hold me back from taking risks, trying new things, or believing in my abilities?)

The Inner Critic Isn't You

What would happen if I stopped listening to my inner critic?
(What might I be able to do or feel if I didn't let these thoughts control me?)

What are some counter-statements or affirmations I can use to challenge my inner critic?

(For example: "I am enough," or "Mistakes are part of growth.")

What would it look like to treat myself with the same kindness and understanding I offer others, even when my inner critic is loud?
(How can you show self-compassion instead of self-judgment?)

Chapter 8:
Letting Go Without Falling Apart

"Anger is easier than the raw pain of grief. But healing begins when you stop running. Acknowledge it. Name it. Feel it. Release it."

Letting go sounds like freedom.

But when your sense of identity is wrapped in pain, performance, or protection, letting go can feel like death.

Letting go can mean:

- Releasing the story that you are unworthy.
- Dropping the need to prove yourself through achievement.
- Surrendering the belief that you're responsible for everyone else's emotions.
- Loosening your grip on the past, even if it's what shaped you.
- Saying goodbye to anger, even if it was the only thing shielding you from grief.

And here's the hard truth:

Even when we *want* to heal, we often resist it.

Because healing requires letting go.

And letting go—without knowing who you'll be on the other side—can feel terrifying.

Why We Hold On

We hold on to what hurt us because it gave us something.

A role. A sense of control. A way to cope.

We hold on to the identity of "the strong one" because we're scared to fall apart.

We cling to the belief that we're broken because it's what we've always known.

We carry anger because it's easier than feeling grief.

Letting go doesn't just feel risky—it feels dangerous.

Because when we let go of who we *had* to be, we're left facing who we really are.

And for many of us, that feels like uncharted, unwelcome territory.

Claire's Story: Holding On Too Long

Claire came into therapy because her anger was damaging her relationships at home and at work. She had always considered herself a warm, loving woman—she adored her two young sons and gave everything to her family. But lately, her anger had been erupting with alarming intensity. Her husband was worried. Her colleagues were uncomfortable. And Claire herself was exhausted from carrying the weight of it all.

In therapy, Claire traced the roots of her rage back to a moment frozen in time: the sudden death of her mother when she was only a preteen.

Her mother had been ill, but no one told Claire how serious it was. In her family, death was something you didn't talk about. Claire never got to ask questions, never got to say goodbye, never had the chance to grieve openly. When she tried, she was told to be strong, not to make a fuss, not to upset her father or siblings.

So she buried her grief—and with it, a part of herself.

Over the decades, that buried grief hardened into something else: anger. A sharp edge she carried into adulthood. A shield she used to keep people from seeing how vulnerable she still felt inside. It wasn't until her outbursts began to threaten the very relationships she cherished that she finally sought help.

In therapy, Claire began to understand that her anger had been protecting her.

It had kept her from feeling the raw pain of losing her mother.

It had helped her feel powerful when she had once felt helpless.

But that protection had come at a cost.

It kept her stuck in survival mode, always bracing, always controlling, always reacting.

Letting go of her anger meant facing what was underneath: sorrow, fear, longing.

It meant grieving the loss she had never been allowed to grieve.

It meant letting go of the part of her identity that said: *You can't fall apart. You have to hold it all together.*

Claire feared that if she let go of the anger, she'd unravel.

But slowly, with support, she learned that letting go didn't mean breaking down.

It meant breaking *open*.

Letting Go Without Falling Apart

Letting go doesn't mean erasing the past.

It means loosening your grip on the beliefs and behaviors that no longer serve you.

It means:
- You can grieve without crumbling.
- You can surrender without losing yourself.
- You can soften without becoming weak.
- You can release the roles you played—and still be whole.

Your pain shaped you, yes. But it doesn't have to define you forever.

You are allowed to let go of the armor.

You are allowed to put down the weight.

You are allowed to be someone new.

Tip Box: Signs You're Afraid to Let Go

Letting go can feel threatening—especially if your identity is wrapped in performance, control, or pain. Here are some signs you may be resisting release:

1. You fear change more than discomfort.
Even if something hurts, it feels safer than the unknown.

2. You define yourself by your pain.
You're not sure who you are without the wound, the role, or the struggle.

3. You feel guilty when you start to feel better.
Healing feels like betrayal—to your past, to those who hurt you, or to the version of you who suffered.

4. You replay old stories even when new ones are available.
You stay loyal to beliefs that once protected you but now limit you.

5. You equate letting go with weakness or failure.
You fear that if you stop fighting, you'll fall apart completely.

A Gentle Reminder

Letting go isn't the end. It's the beginning.

Of breathing again.

Of feeling again.

Of living in a way that doesn't require constant defense.

You won't fall apart. You'll fall into truth.

And from that truth, you'll rise.

Reflection Questions: Letting Go

These questions aim to help someone confront the emotional attachment they may have to past pain and the fears that keep them from healing. It encourages reflection on what they might gain by releasing that hurt and how it could positively impact their future.

What is the most painful memory I still carry with me, and how does it affect my daily life?

_____
_____
_____
_____
_____
_____
_____
_____
_____
_____
_____
_____
_____
_____
_____

What would it feel like to release the emotional weight of this past hurt? What do I fear would happen if I let go of it?

If I were to forgive (myself/others) for this hurt, what would change in my life? How might I feel different?

What do I believe I am holding onto by keeping this pain alive in my heart? (For example: a sense of control, justice, or protection)

How does holding on to past hurts serve me, and what am I gaining from keeping the pain?

What do I imagine will happen if I completely let go of this pain? Will I lose part of who I am, or would I find freedom?

What do I think might happen to my relationships if I let go of my resentment or hurt toward others?

How would my life be different if I chose to heal and move forward instead of holding on to the past?

What am I afraid of losing if I forgive or release my attachment to past pain?

If I could speak to the part of me that is scared to let go of the past, what would I say to reassure myself?

Chapter 9:
Self-Compassion, Rest, and Setting Boundaries

"Boundaries are a form of self-respect, not selfishness. Saying 'no' to others is saying 'yes' to yourself."

For so long, you've carried the weight-of being the strong one.

The fixer.

The one who holds it together.

You've run on empty—surviving, performing, producing—because rest felt dangerous.

Like if you stopped, everything would fall apart.

Or worse—you'd have to feel what you've been pushing down for years.

Or even worse-you wouldn't be worthy or valuable.

But here's what most people never say out loud:

Healing requires rest, contemplation and self-reflection.

It requires gentleness.

It requires a level of self-compassion most of us were never taught to give ourselves.

You can't hate yourself into wholeness.

You can't shame yourself into change.

And you can't heal when you're constantly in survival mode.

Self-Compassion: The Healing You Were Never Taught

Self-compassion is not indulgence.

It's not weakness.

It's not letting yourself off the hook.

Self-compassion is the brave, quiet decision to stop abandoning yourself.

It's treating your own pain with the same tenderness you'd offer a hurting child.

It's giving yourself permission to feel—to grieve, to breathe, to rest—without guilt.

It's choosing to believe you are worthy of care, even when you don't feel like it.

Most importantly, it's learning to tell yourself the truth:

You were never the problem.

You were never too much.

You were just too alone in what you were carrying.

A Return to Heather's Story: Releasing the Shame

Heather came to therapy with a deeply rooted belief that she was not good enough.

She blamed herself for the chaos of her childhood—for her parents' emotional instability and for being placed with cold, unloving foster homes where she never felt wanted.

In her mind, the narrative was clear:

"If I had been better, quieter, easier, maybe they would have kept me. Maybe they would have loved me."

That belief had shaped her entire life.

It affected how she showed up in relationships.

How she pushed herself at work.

How she held back in moments of joy—never quite believing she deserved it.

But therapy gave Heather something she'd never had before: space to question the story.

As she began to tell the truth—not just about what happened, but about how it made her feel—she started to see things differently.

She realized her parents' failures weren't hers to carry.

She wasn't responsible for their inability to give her a safe, loving home.

And with that realization came release.

Week by week, session by session, Heather gave herself permission to feel what she had buried:

The grief.

The rage.

The loneliness.

The shame.

She cried. She raged. She wept for the little girl who never got to rest.

And then, finally, something shifted.

She exhaled.

She rested.

Not just physically, but emotionally.

For the first time in her life, Heather no longer felt like she had to earn her right to exist.

She was allowed to feel peace.

She was allowed to say no.

She was allowed to set boundaries that protected her energy, her healing, and her worth.

Heather's healing journey wasn't a linear line. She encountered peaks of enlightenment and valleys of grief. But she slowly reached a place where she spent more times in her peaks and less time in her valleys.

Why We Resist Rest

Many people don't resist healing—they resist rest.

Because rest requires trust.

It requires slowing down long enough to hear what your heart is saying.

And for many of us, that voice is filled with grief.

Rest is where the feelings rise.

Rest is where the stories surface.

Rest is where the self-critic gets louder—until we learn to replace it with self-compassion.

If you grew up in a home where love was conditional, where safety was scarce, or where your needs were ignored, you may have internalized this belief:

I have to be doing something to be okay.

I have to be helping, achieving, proving, perfecting—or I'm not worthy and I don't deserve to rest.

But that's a lie your nervous system absorbed to survive.

You are worthy of rest because you are human.

Not because you earned it.

Not because you did enough.

Just because you *are*.

Boundaries as Compassion

To truly rest, you must learn to protect your peace.

That's where boundaries come in.

Boundaries are not walls—they are filters.

They are the way you teach others how to treat you and how you care for yourself.

Rest isn't just about taking a nap.

It's about saying:

- "No, I can't take that on."
- "I need space to process."
- "I'm not available to be the emotional dumping ground today."
- "I matter too."

Setting boundaries is an act of self-compassion.

It allows your healing to deepen without being constantly disrupted by the needs, expectations, or dysfunction of others.

Setting boundaries when you're not accustomed to doing so can be frightening. "What if she gets mad at me?" "What if I get rejected?" "What if I don't get invited again?"

If this **catastrophic thinking** comes to fruition, what does that tell you about the quality of the relationship and the respect and concern for your wellbeing?

To level up the quality of your life, you have to level up the quality of your relationships.

Tip Box: What Self-Compassion Might Look Like Today

- Saying no without over explaining
- Letting yourself cry without shame
- Eating when you're hungry rather than feeding everyone else first
- Taking a nap and calling it sacred, not lazy
- Stopping when your body says stop—even if your to-do list isn't done
- Speaking to yourself like someone you love
- Setting boundaries without guilt

A Gentle Reminder

Rest is not quitting.

Compassion is not weakness.

Boundaries are not rejection.

They are the soft, steady choices of someone who is finally learning to heal.

You don't have to prove anything anymore.

You don't have to carry what was never yours.

You don't have to hustle to be loved.

You are allowed to rest.

Reflection Questions: Self-Compassion and Rest

These questions are designed to encourage reflection on how over-functioning and over-achieving affect a person's well-being, while also helping them explore practical ways to practice self-compassion and set healthy boundaries.

When was the last time I pushed myself too hard to achieve something, and how did it impact my physical and emotional well-being?

What are the signs that I am over-functioning or taking on too much responsibility? How do I feel when I'm doing this?

What would it look like to treat myself with the same kindness and care I show to others, especially when I'm overwhelmed?

What does "enough" look like for me in terms of effort, productivity, and achievement? How can I remind myself that I don't need to be perfect to be worthy?

How can I practice saying "no" in a way that feels empowering rather than guilty or selfish? What would it feel like to set a boundary with someone I'm afraid to disappoint?

What are some small ways I can show myself compassion when I fail or make a mistake, rather than criticizing or punishing myself?

How do I feel when I take a break or step back from responsibilities? How can I embrace rest as an essential part of being productive, rather than a luxury I don't deserve?

What are my personal limits when it comes to work, helping others, and taking on new tasks? How can I communicate those limits clearly and confidently to others?

How can I celebrate my progress and achievements, even the small ones, without needing to do more or be perfect?

What would it look like to create a daily or weekly practice of self-compassion and boundary-setting, and how can I begin today?

Chapter 10:
You Were Never Broken

If you've made it this far, take a breath.

Let yourself feel the weight of what you've just walked through.

You've revisited painful stories.

You've questioned old beliefs.

You've named what was once unspoken.

And maybe, for the first time, you've started to see yourself with more clarity—and more compassion.

This work is not easy.

But it's the most important work there is.

Because here's the truth:

You were never broken.

You were wounded.

You were left to carry what wasn't yours.

You were shaped by pain, not defined by it.

And now, you're learning that healing isn't about becoming someone new.

It's about returning to the self you were always meant to be—before the shame, before the lies, before the armor.

You are not your trauma.

You are not your anxious thoughts.

You are not your roles, your past mistakes, or your inner critic.

You are human.

And you are whole—even if you're still healing.

A New Way Forward

As you move forward, remember:

- Your feelings are valid.
- Your pain makes sense.
- And your healing is possible—even if it's not linear.

There will be days when the old beliefs resurface. That's okay.

You're not doing it wrong—you're just doing the work.

Keep going.

Keep resting.

Keep rewriting the story.

The Resilient Woman's Circle

You don't have to keep holding it all in.

You don't have to carry it alone.

And you don't have to be perfect to be worthy of love.
You are already enough.

You are already healing.

And you are already becoming whole.

Afterword — What Happened To...

The case studies I've shared are based on real clients from my private therapy practice. While names and identifying details have been changed to protect anonymity, each story represents the core issues I see most often in my work.

I left some of these stories intentionally unresolved in earlier chapters, but that doesn't feel right now. If I were reading this book, I'd want to know what happened. So here we go...

Chapter 1 – Heather's Story

Heather carried deep and complex emotional wounds. Many of our sessions were spent with her telling and retelling her story through tears. Simply being able to speak her truth felt like a critical step in her healing.

Like my neighbor's cut toe story, Heather had a lot of wound-cleansing to do before she could move forward.

A pivotal shift occurred when she finally understood that she was not to blame for the chaos of her childhood. Realizing that her parents' inability to care for her was the root of her trauma lifted an enormous emotional burden.

Heather became more joyful and lighter in spirit. She learned to set boundaries with others and recognize distorted thinking—especially her tendency to personalize situations that had nothing to do with her.

She eventually made the empowering decision to move closer to one of her sisters, so she wouldn't feel so isolated and alone.

Chapter 2 – Samantha's Secret

After many months of therapy, Samantha shared a painful secret: she had been molested by a close family friend at age nine. Her abuser had threatened her into silence, warning that she'd be taken from her family if she told anyone.

As illogical as it sounds, Samantha internalized the belief that the abuse was her fault. She thought she had to be perfect to protect herself and her family. But the weight of the secret, coupled with the constant pressure to be flawless, eventually became unbearable.

Because the perpetrator had passed away and Samantha didn't want to upset her elderly parents, she chose not to tell them. She did, however, take steps to unburden herself in other ways. Though she considered leaving her high-pressure job, she realized she actually loved her work—just not the unsustainable workload. After a candid conversation with her firm's partners, they reduced her caseload and brought in another paralegal to support her.

Samantha is slowly learning that she doesn't need to be everything to everyone to be worthy of love. With a more balanced schedule, she's discovering the value of simply being present with her family—without needing to prove her love through gifts or achievements.

Chapter 3 – Angela's Story

Angela's road to recovery from hypervigilance and perfectionism was long and challenging. She was hardwired to always double-check, stay alert, and avoid mistakes. I gently encouraged her to start making small, inconsequential errors on purpose to break the cycle of fear.

Reluctantly, she agreed. Her first assignment was to arrive five minutes late to work. She was anxious but followed through. And—nothing bad happened. This small act was a major turning point.

Over time, Angela practiced allowing minor imperfections and eventually moved on to the harder task: delegation. Although she hired capable staff for her business, her micromanaging drove them away. We created a progressive plan to help her let go of control and trust her employees. She even shared the plan with her team.

While she still struggles when anxious, Angela has made tremendous progress—she's probably 75% better than when we first began.

Chapter 4 – Lea's Story

Lea's first priority was managing her panic attacks. We began with education, breathing tools, and a referral for medication. Once her nervous system calmed—thanks to an anti-anxiety prescription—she was finally able to focus on deeper healing.

We began addressing the perfectionism and overthinking that had dominated her life. As her confidence grew, so did her world. She slowly re-engaged with the things she once loved—book club, Pilates, even joining a kickball league. These weren't overnight changes, but they marked a steady return to her baseline functioning.

Later, Lea uncovered a painful piece of her past. She learned that her mother had been addicted to drugs, and her father had given her mother an ultimatum: enter rehab or he would file for divorce and seek custody. Her mother chose to leave.

Lea had minimal and inconsistent contact with her mother throughout childhood. As of our last session, she still didn't know where her mother lived. But despite this loss, Lea was learning how to nurture herself in ways her mother couldn't.

Chapter 5 – Blair's Story

When Blair first entered therapy, she offered a stream of rationalizations for why she had stolen from her employer. She insisted she wasn't paid enough, that her boss had plenty of money and wouldn't miss it, and that "everyone does it" — all her friends steal too. While she acknowledged that it was technically wrong, she added bluntly, "It was only wrong because I got caught." With a cavalier attitude, she even admitted she would probably do it again.

But as trust began to form in the therapeutic space, a different version of Blair slowly emerged — a hurt, vulnerable little girl who had been deeply wounded by her mother's favoritism toward her sister and the harsh judgment directed at her. Blair longed for a close, loving connection with her mother — the kind of bond her sister seemed to enjoy effortlessly. Instead, she was met with rejection, exclusion, and a sense of never being good enough.

Week after week, Blair returned to these early wounds, crying as she finally gave voice to the pain she had carried for so long. There was a kind of emotional detox — a clearing out of the shame, grief, and rage that had lived unspoken in her body. As she did this work, something began to shift. She reached a new level of clarity and self-awareness.

Blair came to a decision: although the urge to steal might still tempt her, she no longer wanted to be defined by it. "I don't want 'thief' to be my identity," she said.

More profoundly, she made another choice — to stop chasing her mother's love and approval. It was as if she flipped a switch from *"You hurt me"* to *"Your opinion of me no longer matters."* In that moment, Blair experienced a freedom she had never known. She realized she had been living in a prison built from her own thoughts and the hope that her mother would one day change.

Now, she was ready to build a different life-one defined not by pain or past roles, but by her true self.

Chapter 6 – My Story

In many ways, this book—and the work I've dedicated my life to—represents the arc of my own healing. It took years of searching, struggling, and avoiding before I was ready to turn inward and face the pain I had long carried. But when I finally allowed myself to confront the source of my suffering—what I often call "the belly of the beast"—the real transformation began.

Healing didn't happen overnight. It came slowly, through moments of clarity, grief, release, and growth. I began to see myself not through the lens of what had happened to me, but through the lens of who I truly was beneath the pain.

I still experience anxiety from time to time—but it no longer controls me. I recognize it for what it is: a signal, not a sentence. I have tools to manage it, perspective to understand it, and compassion to meet it without fear. These days, I feel grounded in who I am. I move through life with more self-trust and a quiet confidence in what lies ahead.

Final Reflections

Each of the women in this book remains on her healing journey. Recovery is not a straight line, and their stories are far from complete. But what's changed is that they are no longer defined by their pasts. They are learning, like so many of us, that healing is possible—not by erasing the past, but by reclaiming ourselves.

Acknowledgments

The stories in this book are inspired by the incredible, resilient women I've had the honor of working with over the years. The case studies are real in essence—but let's be clear: names, details, and identifying features have been changed, blurred, or creatively rewritten to protect client confidentiality (and avoid awkward grocery store encounters).

Also, a quick shoutout to artificial intelligence. Yes, I had help. I used AI to clean up my grammar, untangle my sentences, and keep me from writing like a sleep-deprived raccoon. It was like having a very smart, very patient co-writer who never got tired of me saying, "Does this sound okay?"

But the heart of this book? That's all mine. (Okay, and maybe a little bit yours, too.)

To my clients, thank you for trusting me with your stories. And to the reader holding this book: thank you for showing up—for yourself, and for your healing. You are so worth it.

About the Author

Jan Truszkowski, MSW, LICSW, always knew she had a book in her. But like many women who spend their lives helping others, she found it hard to slow down long enough to put her own story on the page—until now.

Her journey into the healing professions began in tragedy: Jan's father was killed when she was just four years old. Like so many drawn to the helping fields in search of their own healing, she pursued a career in Social Work, eventually earning her Master's degree from the University of Kentucky. After many winding career paths, she found her calling in doing for others what once meant so much to her—offering a safe place to be seen, heard, and understood.

Over the years, Jan has listened to thousands of stories filled with pain, anxiety, and self-doubt. Through her work as a therapist, she has provided insight, compassion, and a gentle nudge toward healing. Now in the giving-back phase of life, she's reaching out a hand to women who may not be as far down the trail, but are walking the same road.

When she's not offering therapy or writing, you'll likely find her visiting family, out on the golf course, reading a good book, indulging in a great meal, or watching something wonderfully binge-worthy.